Living With...

ADHD

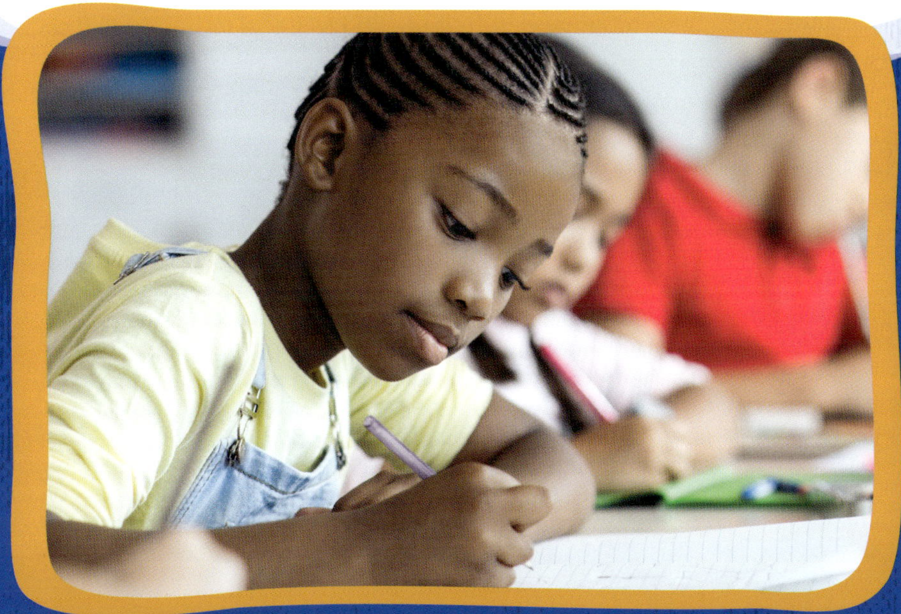

Nancy Dickmann

Consultant: Marjorie Hogan, MD

Brown Bear Books

Published by Brown Bear Books Ltd
4877 N. Circulo Bujia
Tucson, AZ 85718
USA

and

Studio G14, Regent Studios,
1 Thane Villas, London N7 7PH, UK

ISBN 978-1-78121-801-3 (library bound)
ISBN 978-1-78121-807-5 (paperback)

Library of Congress Cataloging-in-Publication Data available on request

Text: Nancy Dickmann
Consultant: Marjorie Hogan, MD, Professor of Pediatrics, University of Minnesota, Retired staff pediatrician, Hennepin Healthcare
Design Manager: Keith Davis
Children's Publisher: Anne O'Daly

Manufactured in the United States of America
CPSIA compliance information: Batch#AG/5651

Picture Credits
The photographs in this book are used by permission and through the courtesy of:

Front Cover: Shutterstock: imtmphoto;
Interior: iStock: Boogich 4-5, fizkes 6, imgorthand 10-11; Shutterstock: Andrew Angelov 16-17, BalanceFormCreative 8-9, Bilanol 22b, Diego Cervo 16, fizkes 14, Edward Indy 12, Anna Mentre 20, NDAB Creativity 14-15, Sergey Novikov 20-21, PHILIPIMAGE 18, Photographee.eu 18-19, Andrey Popov 10, Rido 8, Oksana Ryazanova 22t, Olena Yakobchuk 4, Dmytro Zinkevych 12-13.

All other artwork and photography © Brown Bear Books.

t-top, r-right, l-left, c-center, b-bottom

Brown Bear Books has made every attempt to contact the copyright holder. If you have any information about omissions please contact: licensing@brownbearbooks.co.uk

Websites
The website addresses in this book were valid at the time of going to press. However, it is possible that contents or addresses may change following publication of this book. No responsibility for any such changes can be accepted by the author or the publisher. Readers should be supervised when they access the Internet.

Words in **bold** appear in the Words to Know on page 23.

Contents

What Is ADHD?

Everyone is different. We act in different ways. Some people like to curl up with a good book. Others like to run around and be active. These differences help make us who we are.

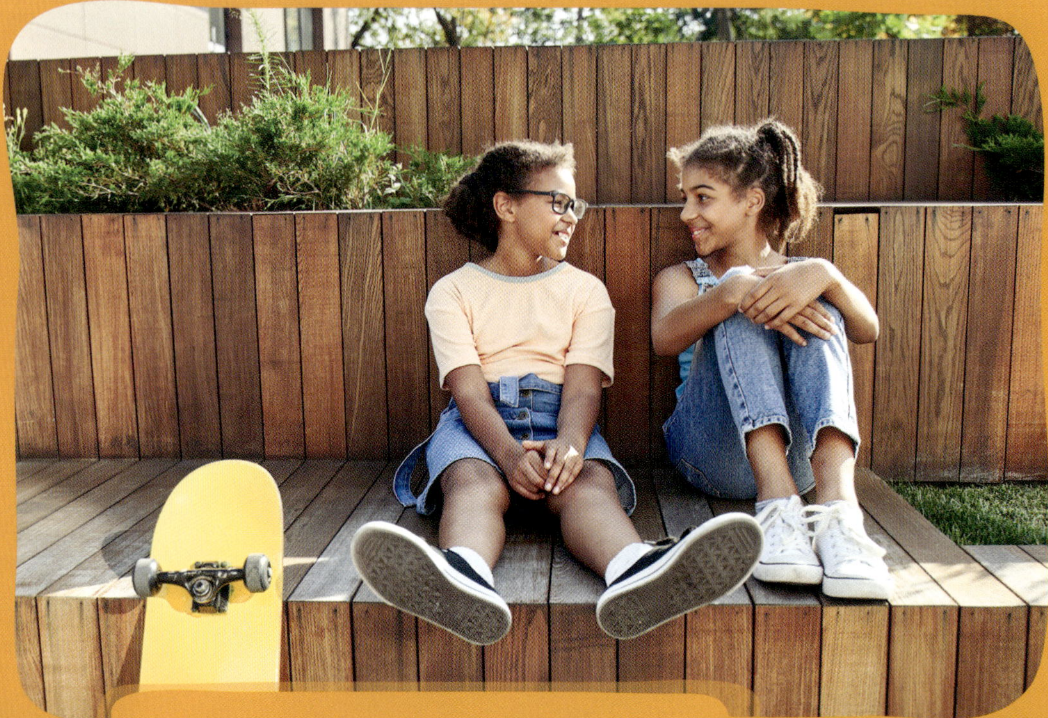

Some people like to talk. Others prefer to listen.

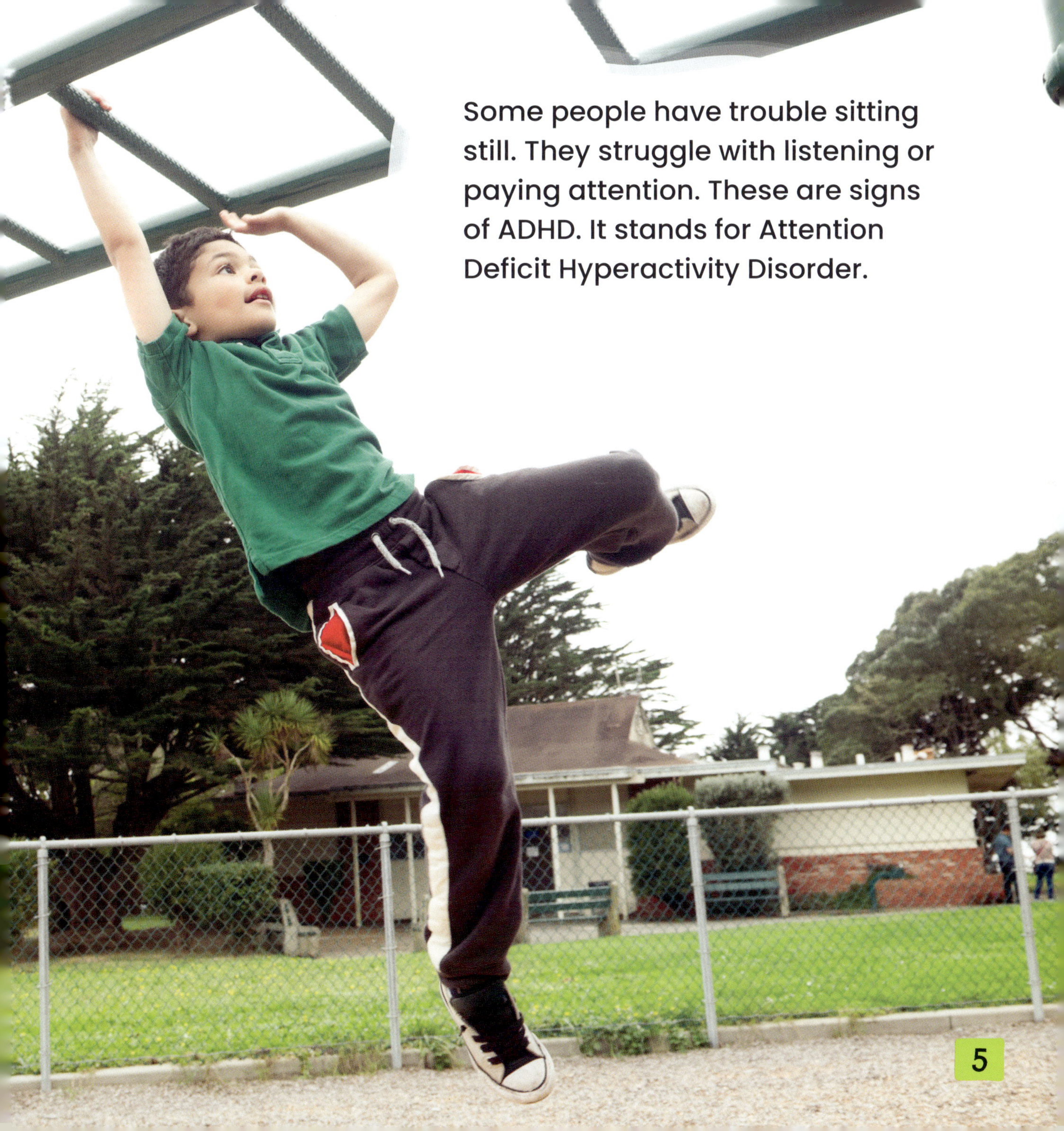

Some people have trouble sitting still. They struggle with listening or paying attention. These are signs of ADHD. It stands for Attention Deficit Hyperactivity Disorder.

Hyperactivity

Most children like to run and play. But some children are hyperactive. They are always on the go. They often act on **impulse**. They can't stop themselves jumping in or saying something.

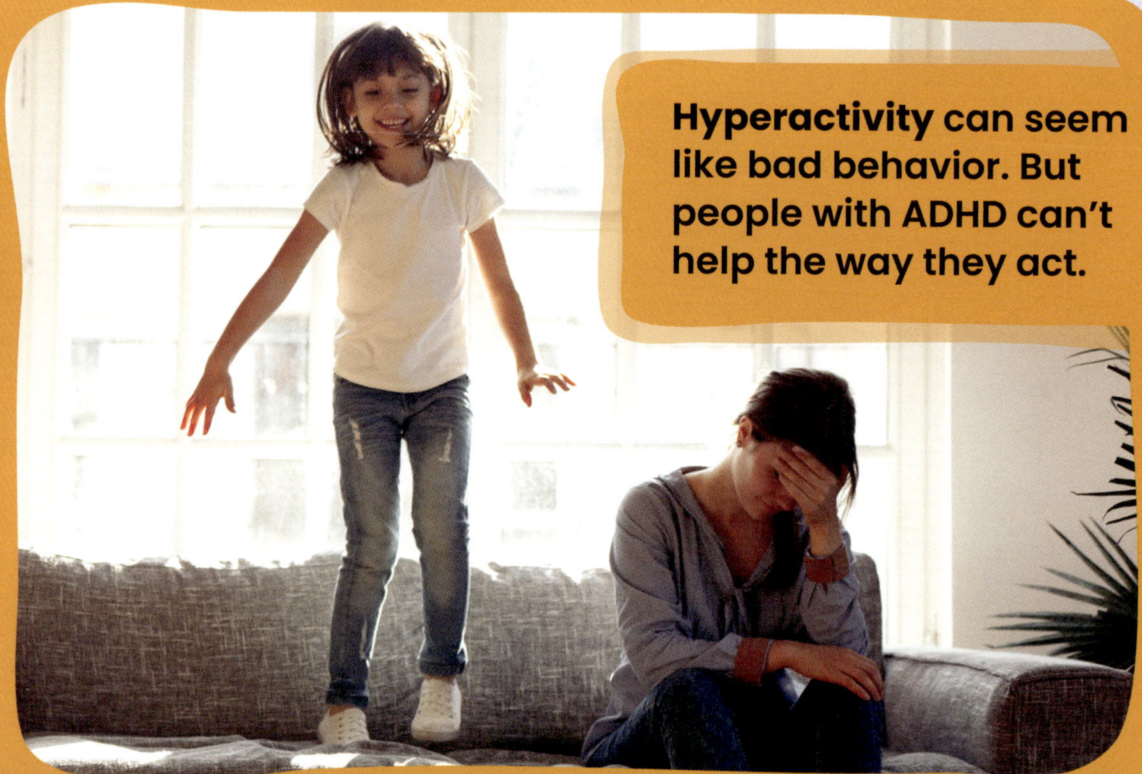

Hyperactivity can seem like bad behavior. But people with ADHD can't help the way they act.

Signs of Hyperactivity and Impulsivity

- Fidgeting and squirming
- Tapping hands or feet
- Running or climbing
- Talking a lot
- Interrupting other people
- Not looking out for danger
- Not waiting for their turn

We all probably do most of these things sometimes. But someone with hyperactivity does them a lot.

Paying Attention

ADHD is a mix of two conditions. One is hyperactivity. The other is attention **deficit**. People with this have a short attention span. They have trouble staying focused. They get distracted easily.

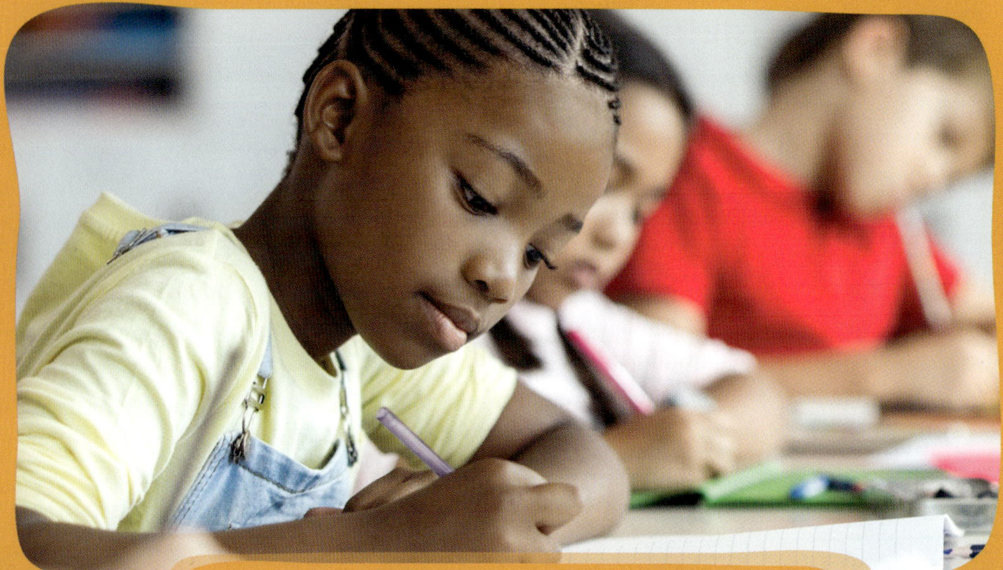

Doing work at school takes focus. People with ADHD often make careless mistakes.

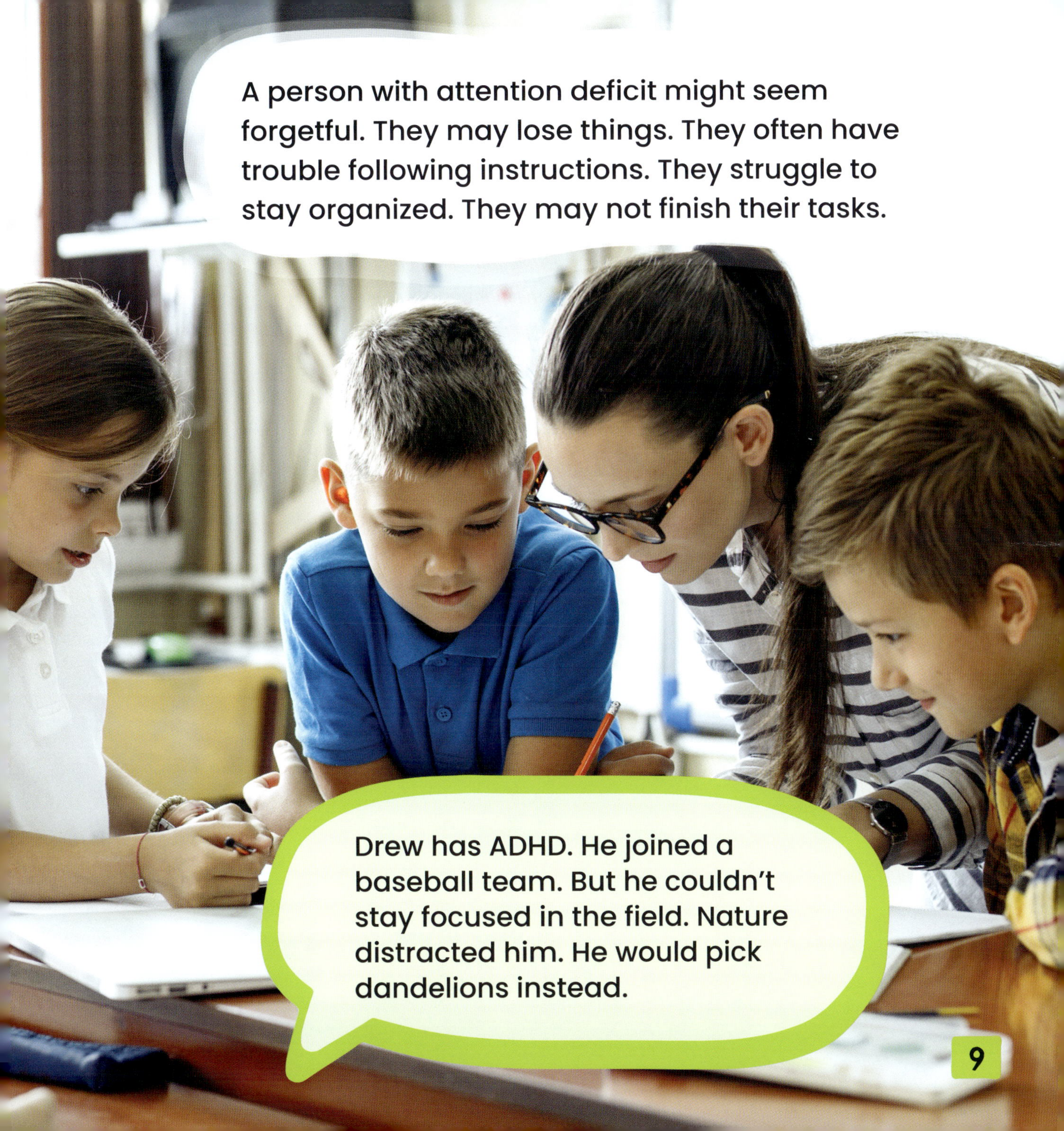

A person with attention deficit might seem forgetful. They may lose things. They often have trouble following instructions. They struggle to stay organized. They may not finish their tasks.

Drew has ADHD. He joined a baseball team. But he couldn't stay focused in the field. Nature distracted him. He would pick dandelions instead.

What's the Problem?

Have you ever watched a boring film? You might start to fidget. ADHD is more than that. The **symptoms** show up at home and at school. They make a person's life harder.

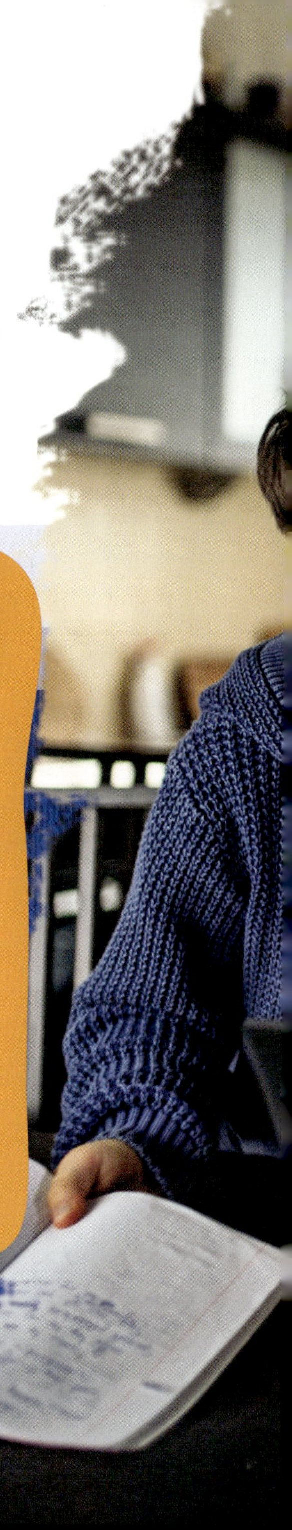

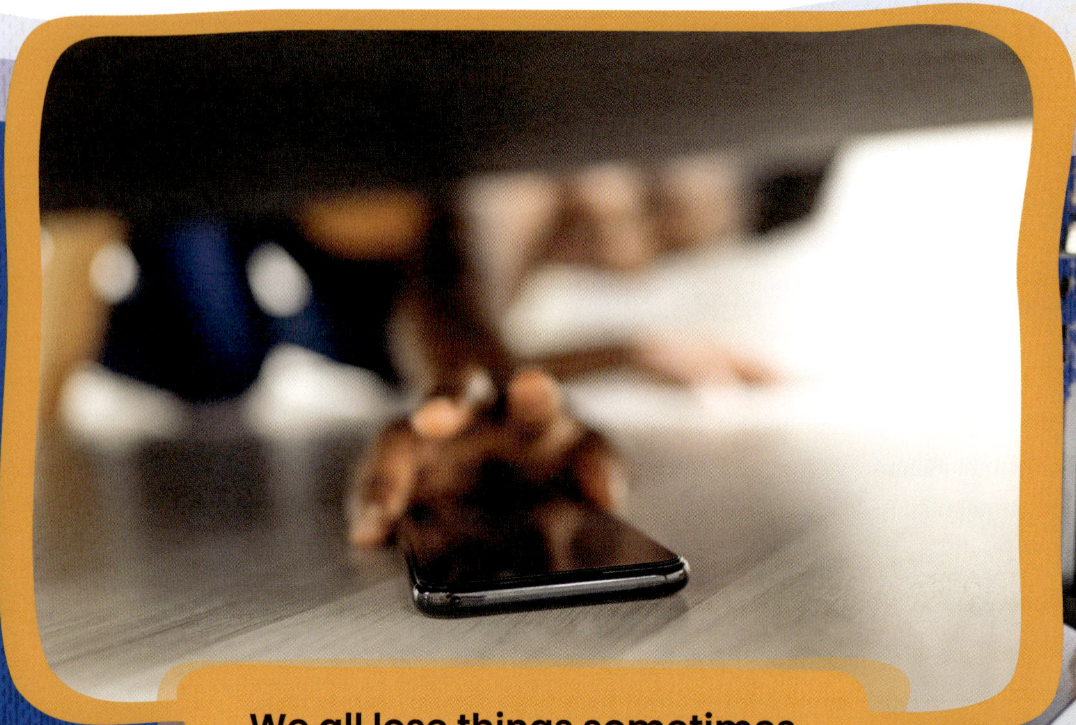

We all lose things sometimes. It doesn't always mean you have ADHD.

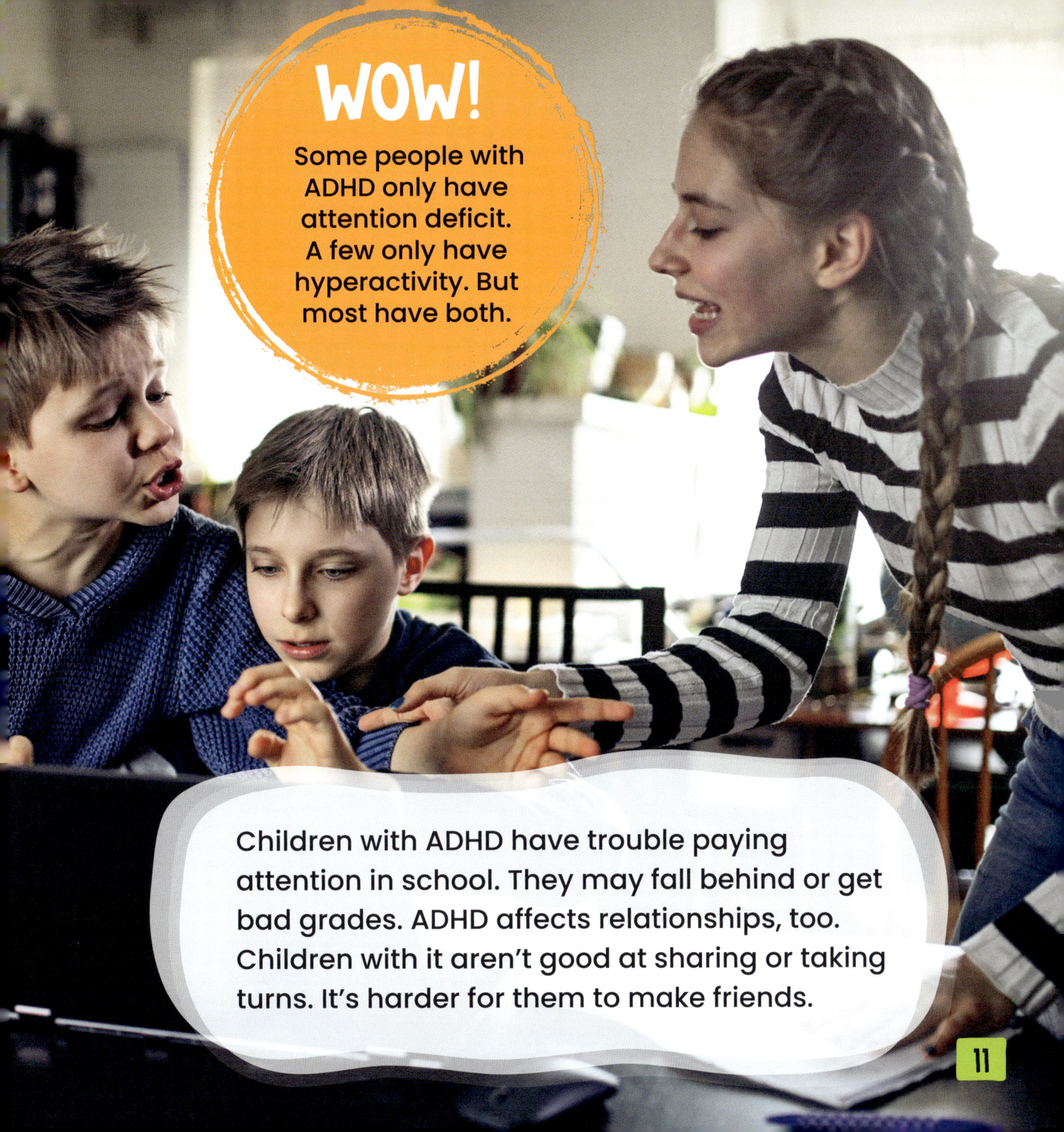

WOW!

Some people with ADHD only have attention deficit. A few only have hyperactivity. But most have both.

Children with ADHD have trouble paying attention in school. They may fall behind or get bad grades. ADHD affects relationships, too. Children with it aren't good at sharing or taking turns. It's harder for them to make friends.

Inside the Brain

Your brain is like a computer. It runs your body! It controls breathing and moving. It controls learning and remembering. ADHD has to do with the way it grows and develops.

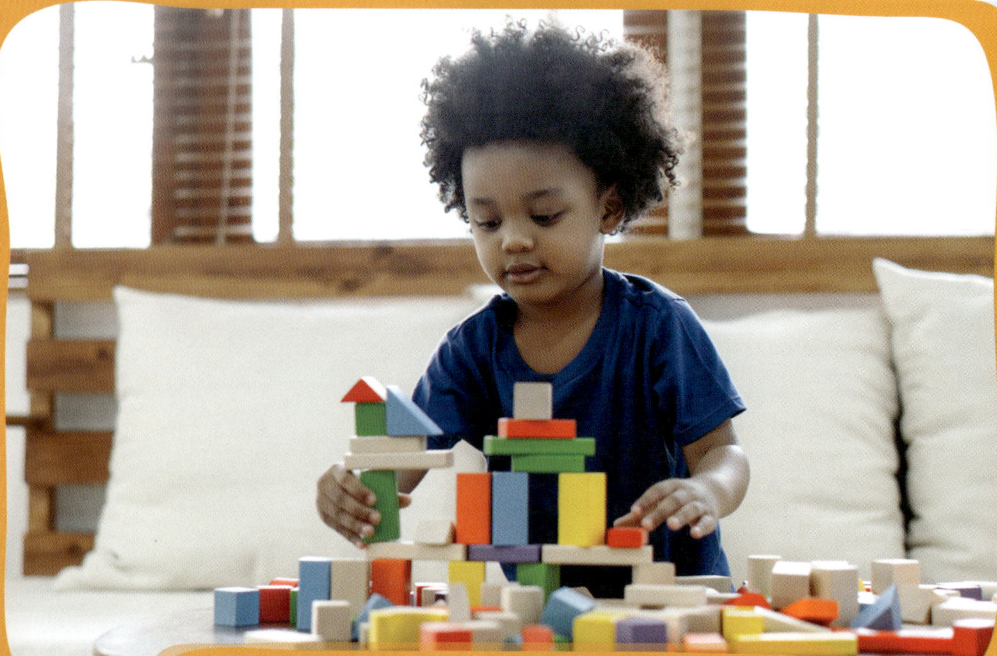

Young children learn quickly. Their brains make new connections as they learn.

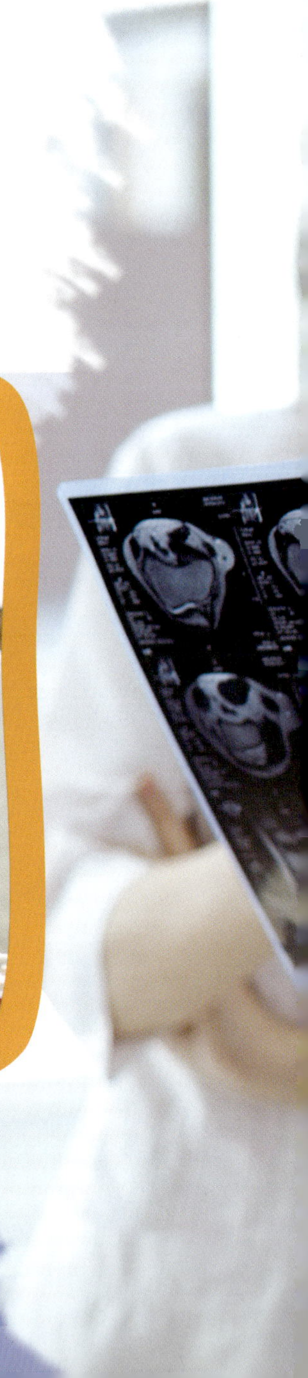

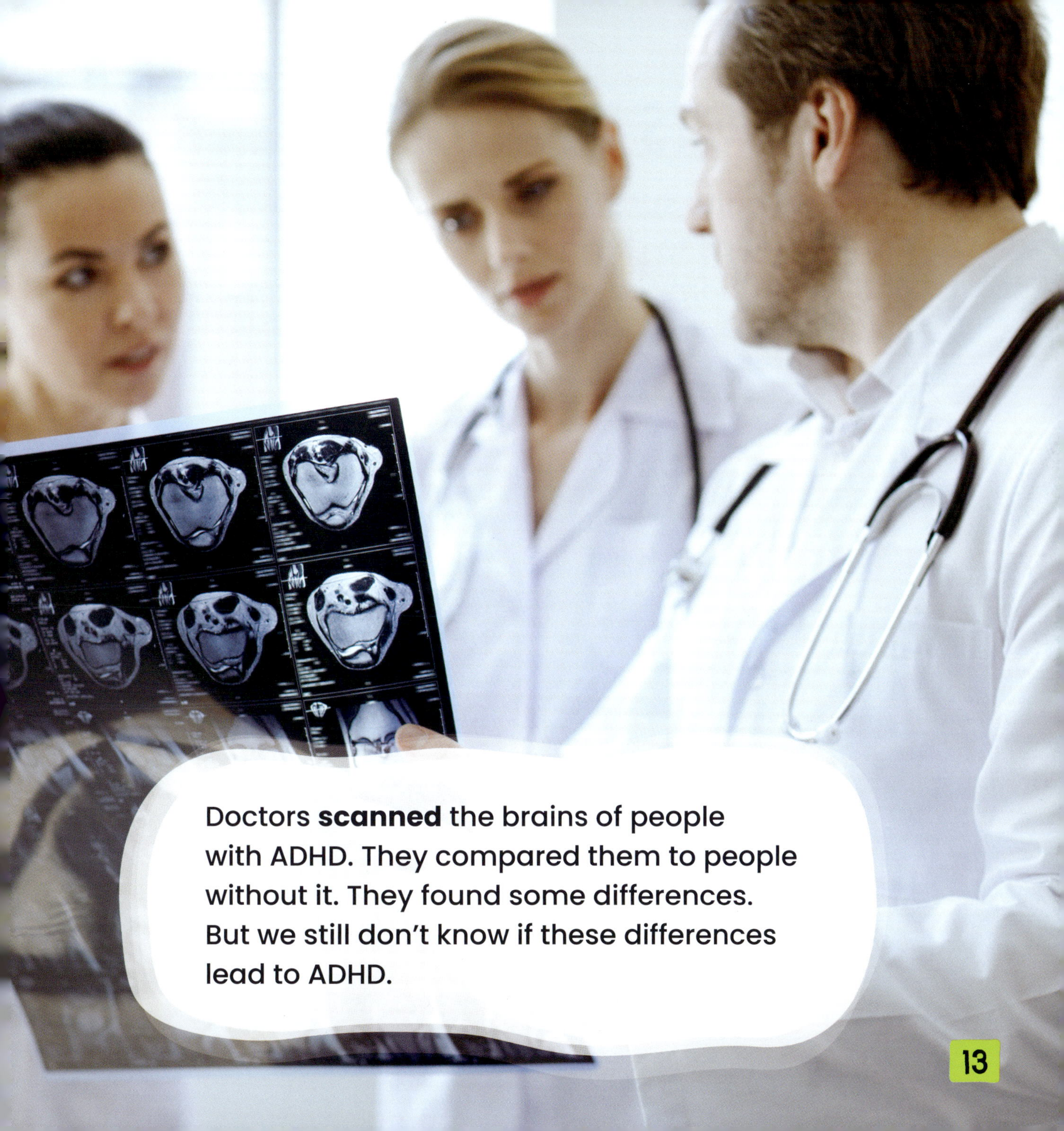

Doctors **scanned** the brains of people with ADHD. They compared them to people without it. They found some differences. But we still don't know if these differences lead to ADHD.

Who Gets ADHD?

No one is quite sure why some people have ADHD. It tends to run in families. Some babies are born too early. They are more at risk. A head injury might also put you at risk.

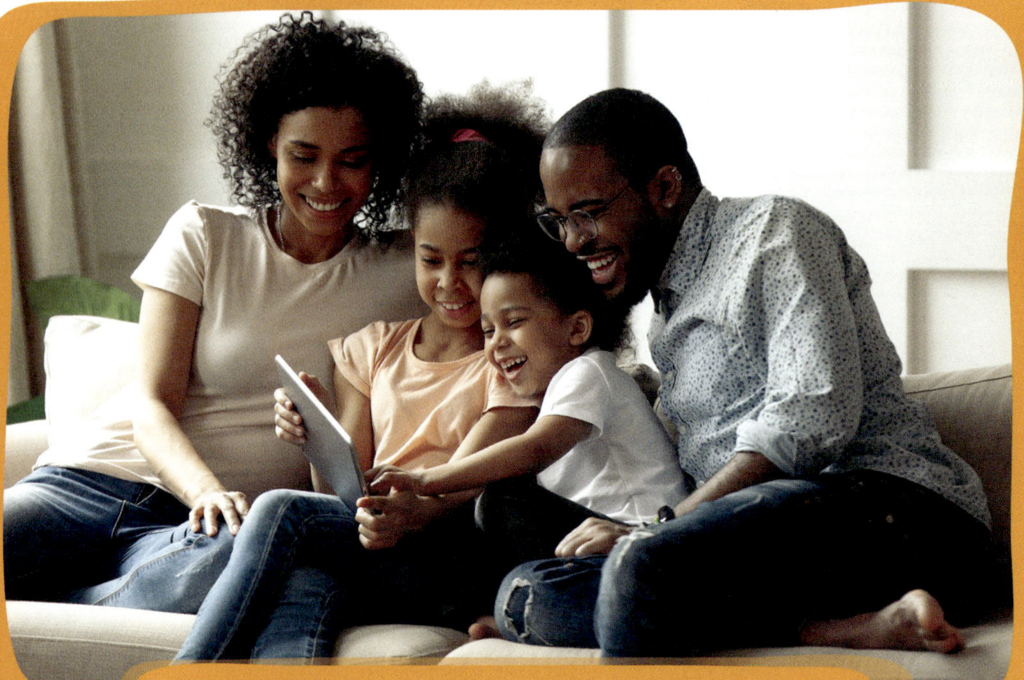

Does your parent have ADHD? Or a brother or sister? That makes you more likely to have it.

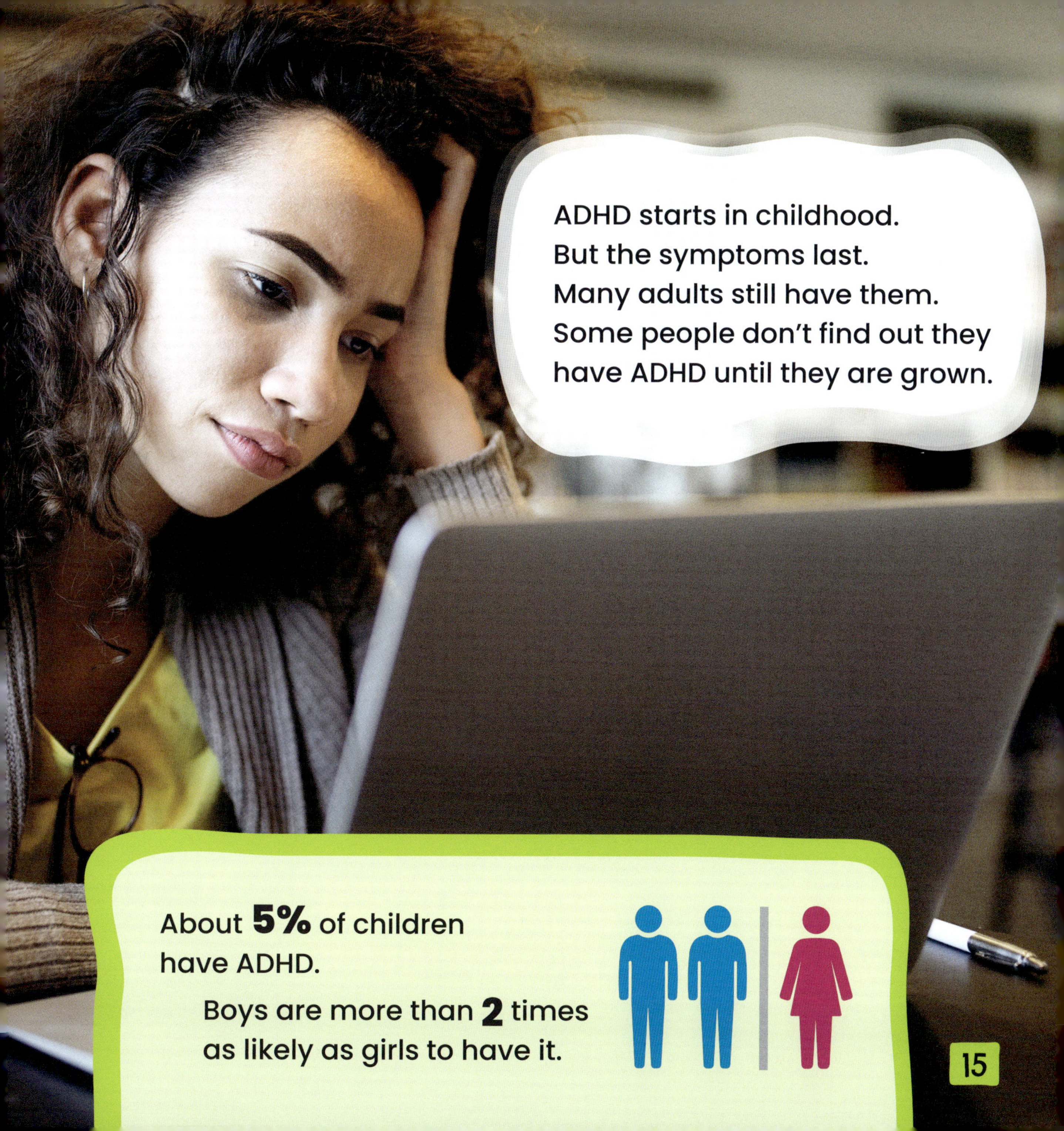

ADHD starts in childhood. But the symptoms last. Many adults still have them. Some people don't find out they have ADHD until they are grown.

About **5%** of children have ADHD.

Boys are more than **2** times as likely as girls to have it.

Testing for ADHD

ADHD is not caused by germs. You can't spot it with a blood test. Instead, doctors look at your symptoms. Some of them can be caused by many things. It's not always ADHD.

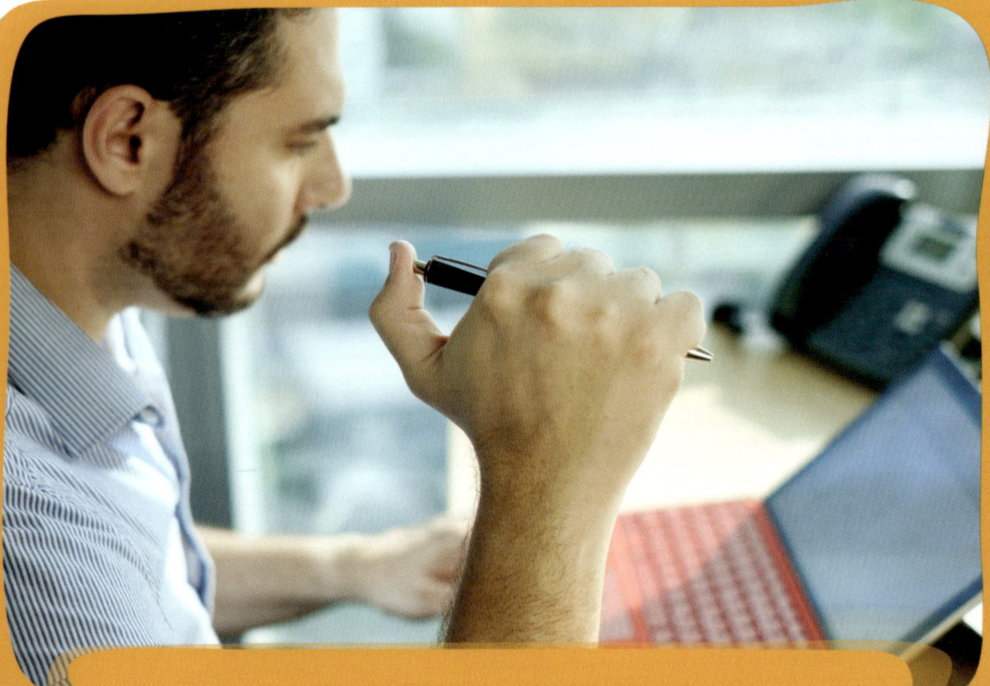

Some people have **anxiety**. It is different from ADHD. But they often fidget too.

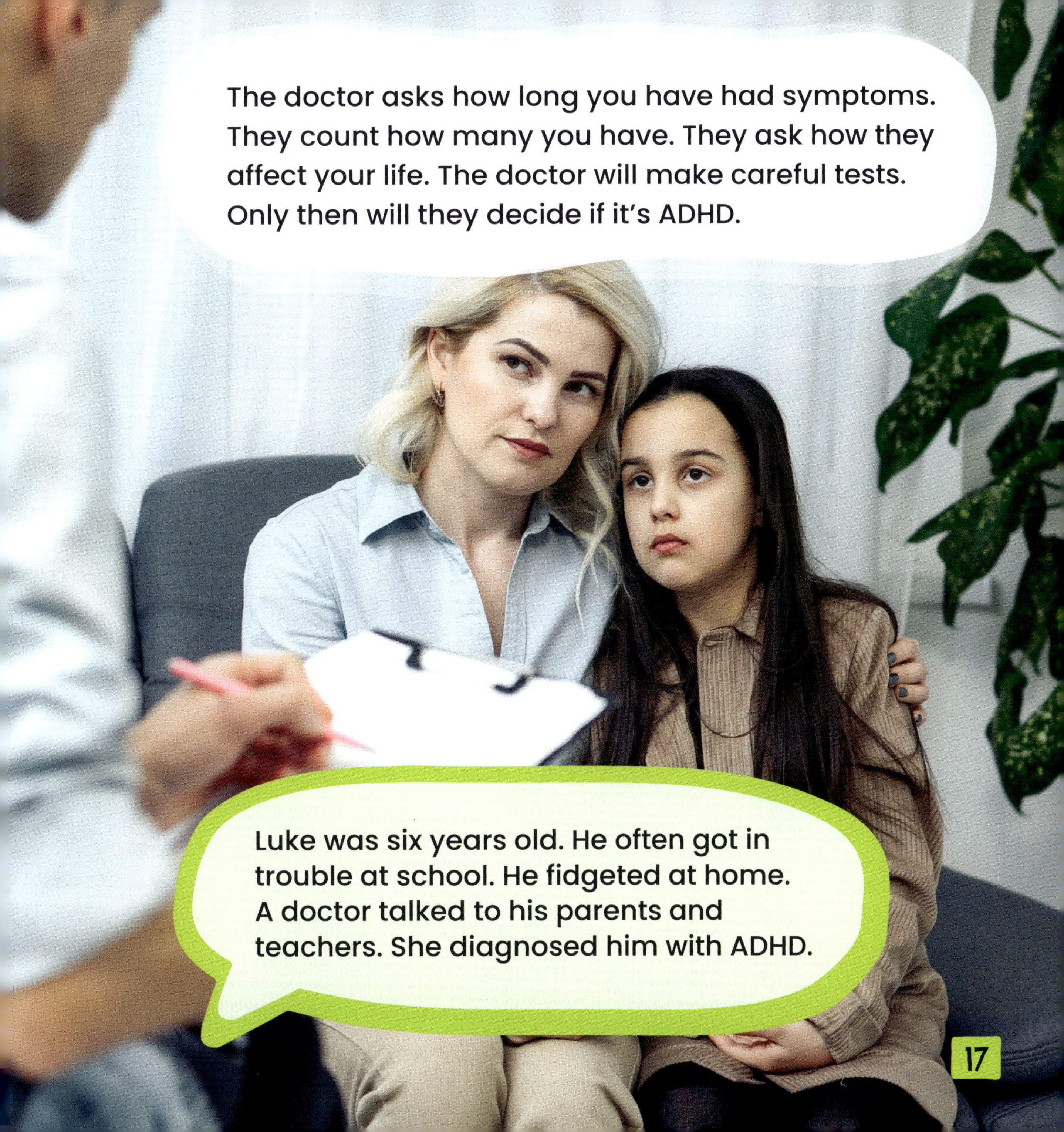

The doctor asks how long you have had symptoms. They count how many you have. They ask how they affect your life. The doctor will make careful tests. Only then will they decide if it's ADHD.

Luke was six years old. He often got in trouble at school. He fidgeted at home. A doctor talked to his parents and teachers. She diagnosed him with ADHD.

Treatments

Some people take medicine for ADHD. Medicine can't cure it. But it can make the symptoms easier to deal with. Medicine helps people concentrate better. It helps them feel calmer.

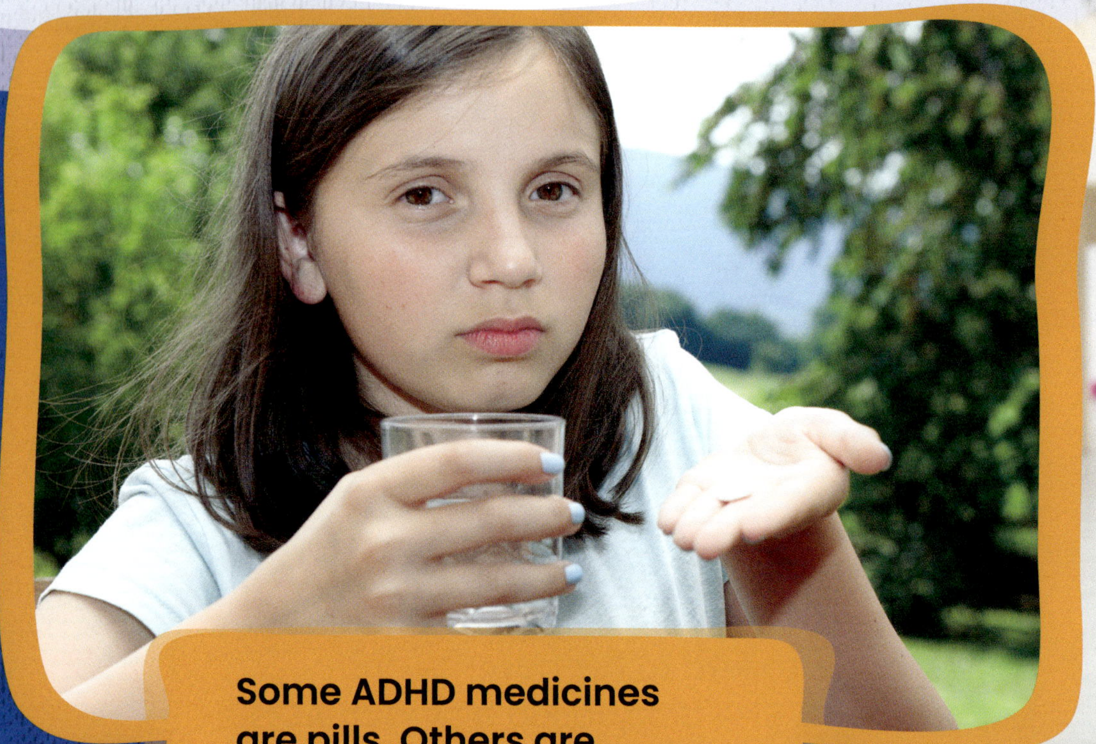

Some ADHD medicines are pills. Others are liquids. You drink them.

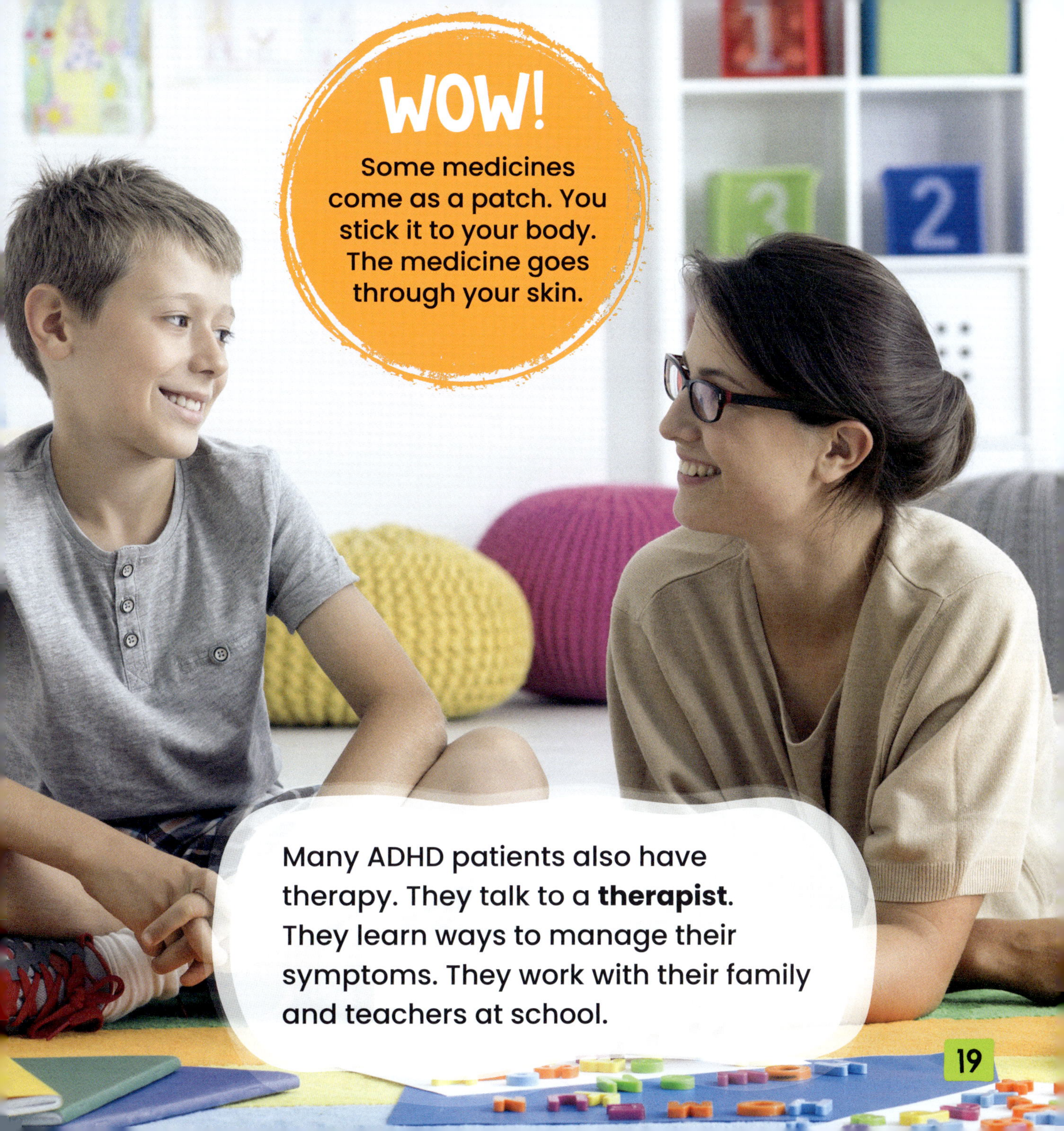

WOW!

Some medicines come as a patch. You stick it to your body. The medicine goes through your skin.

Many ADHD patients also have therapy. They talk to a **therapist**. They learn ways to manage their symptoms. They work with their family and teachers at school.

Living with ADHD

Having a routine helps people with ADHD. They know what to expect. They know what to do. They deal best with short, brief instructions. Rules and rewards can help, too.

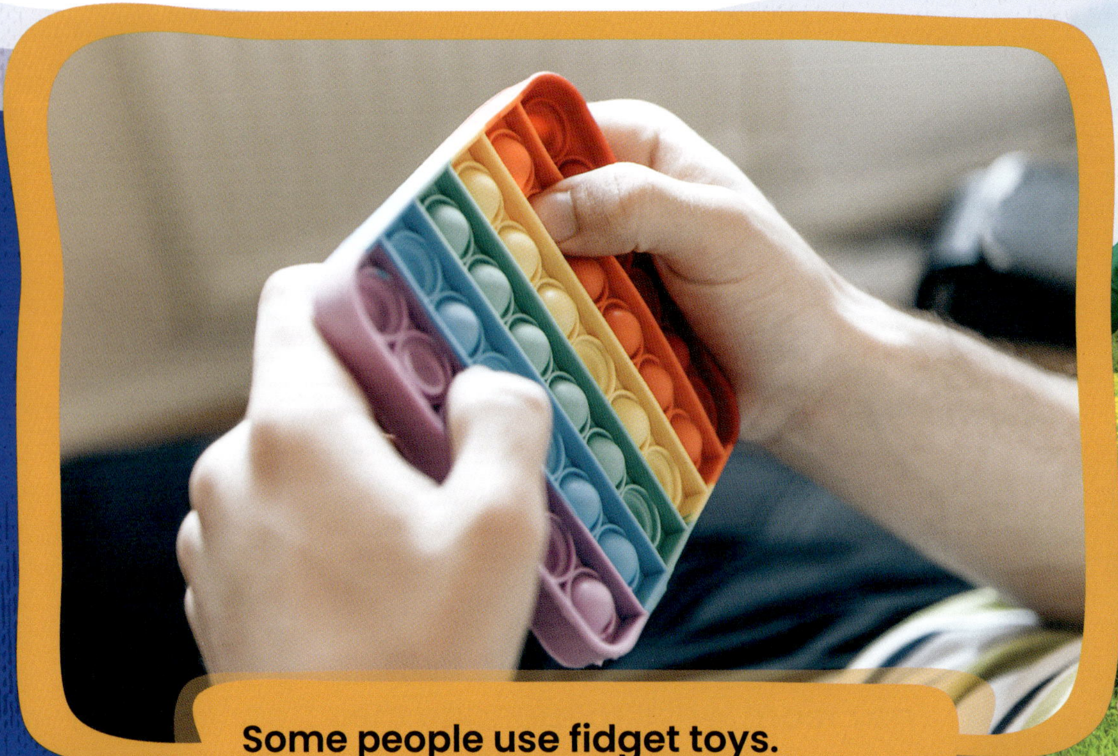

Some people use fidget toys. These keep their hands busy. This helps them concentrate.

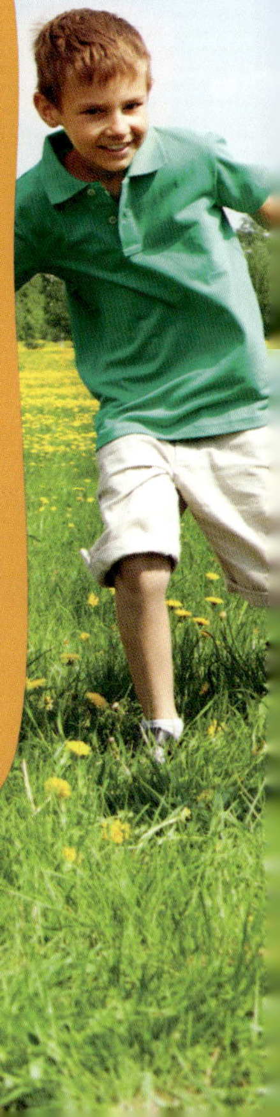

Do you know someone with ADHD? Be patient with them. ADHD symptoms sometimes look like bad behavior. But children with ADHD can't help the way they act. Make sure they feel accepted.

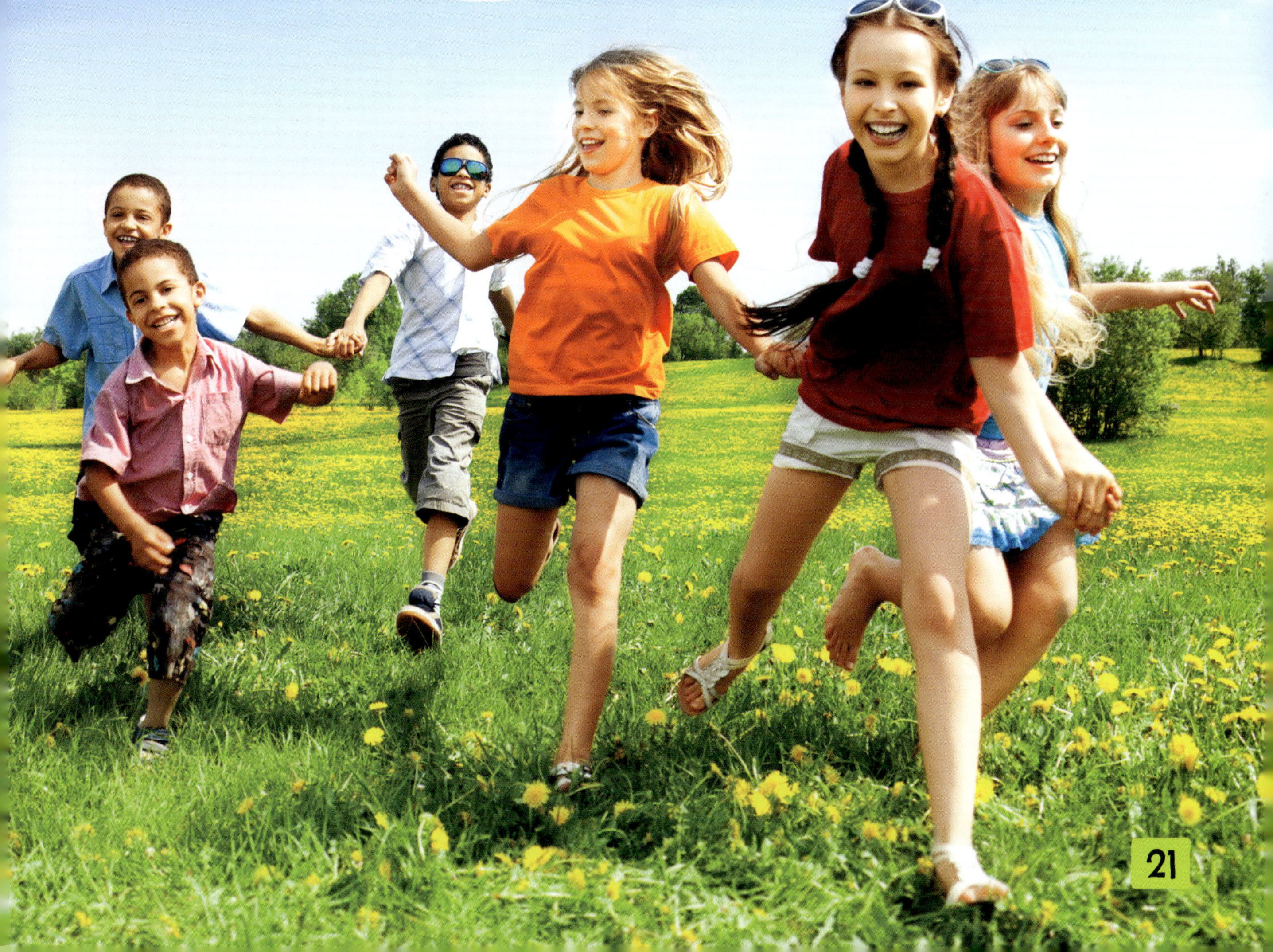

Activity

People with ADHD often meditate. It helps them stay calm and focused. Anyone can meditate! It's good for dealing with stress or worries.

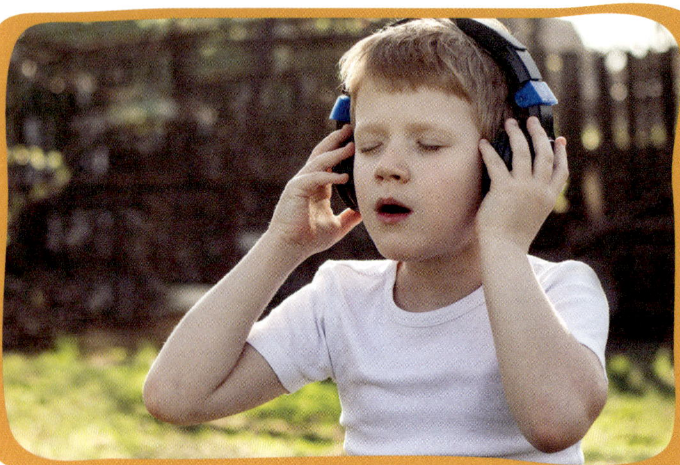

Find a quiet place. Sit in a comfortable pose. (If you're happier walking around, that's fine too!) Put on some quiet, gentle music.

Take a slow, deep breath in. Notice how it makes your body feel. Then breathe out, nice and slow. Keep it up until you feel calm.

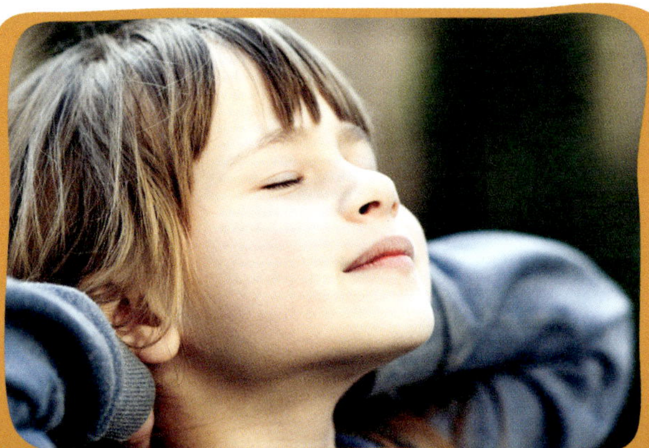

Words to Know

anxiety a medical condition where people worry or feel nervous a lot

deficit a lack of something, or not having enough

hyperactivity behavior that is constantly active and sometimes disruptive

impulse a sudden strong urge to do something

scanned used technology to take a detailed picture of the inside of something

symptoms the outward signs of an illness, such as a fever or rash

therapist a person who is trained to listen to a person and help them deal with their problems

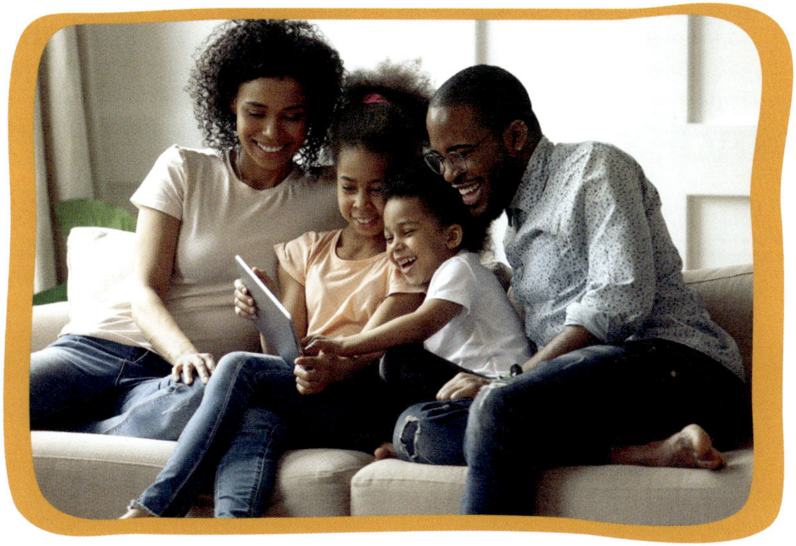

Find out More

Websites

cdc.gov/ncbddd/kids/adhd.html#school

dkfindout.com/us/human-body/brain-and-nerves/brain/

kidshealth.org/en/kids/adhdkid.html

Books

A Book About ADHD (Healthy Minds)
Holly Duhig, Rosen Publishing, 2020

Understanding ADHD
Jessica Rusick, ABDO Books, 2022

Your Brain Is Amazing: How the Human Mind Works
Esperanza Habinger, Orca Book Publishers, 2023

Index